# Plant Based Sweet Wonders

AF394457

Tasty and Incredibly Healthy Desserts to Enjoy

Your Diet and Lose Weight

Tanya Lang

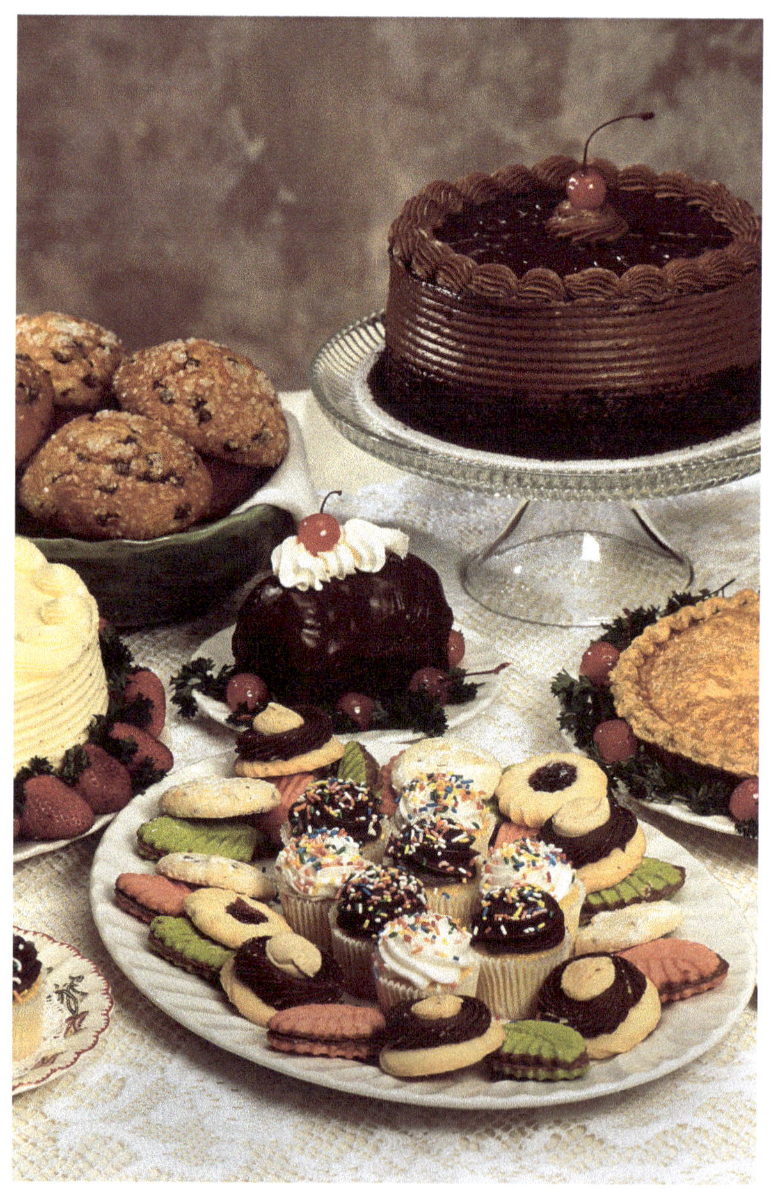

© **Copyright 2021 - All rights reserved.**

The content contained within this book may not be reproduced, duplicated or transmitted without direct written permission from the author or the publisher.

Under no circumstances will any blame or legal responsibility be held against the publisher, or author, for any damages, reparation, or monetary loss due to the information contained within this book. Either directly or indirectly.

**Legal Notice:**

This book is copyright protected. This book is only for personal use. You cannot amend, distribute, sell, use, quote or paraphrase any part, or the content within this book, without the consent of the author or publisher.

**Disclaimer Notice:**

Please note the information contained within this document is for educational and entertainment purposes only. All effort has been executed to present accurate, up to date, and reliable, complete information. No warranties of any kind are declared or implied. Readers acknowledge that the author is not engaging in the rendering of legal, financial, medical or professional advice. The content within this book has been derived from various sources. Please consult a licensed professional before attempting any techniques outlined in this book.

By reading this document, the reader agrees that under no circumstances is the author responsible for any losses, direct or indirect, which are incurred as a result of the use of information contained within this document, including, but not limited to, — errors, omissions, or inaccuracies.

# TABLE OF CONTENT

# Coconut Chocolate Cake

• Preparation Time: 10 minutes | Cooking Time: 30 minutes | Servings:  12

Ingredients:

 • 4 tablespoons flaxseed mixed with 5 tablespoons water

 • 1 cup coconut flesh, unsweetened and shredded

 • 1 teaspoon vanilla extract

 • 2 tablespoons cocoa powder

 • 1 teaspoon baking soda

 • 2 cups almond flour

 • 4 tablespoons stevia

 • 2 tablespoons lime zest

 • 2 cups coconut cream

Directions:

• In a bowl, combine the flax meal with the coconut, the vanilla, and the other ingredients, whisk well and transfer to a cake pan.

• Cook the cake at 360 degrees F for 30 minutes, cool down, and serve.

Nutrition:

• Calories 268, Fat 23.9, Fiber 5.1, Carbs 9.4, Protein 6.1

# Mint Chocolate Cream

Preparation Time: 10 minutes | Cooking Time: 0 minutes | Servings: 6

Ingredients:

- 1 cup coconut oil, melted
- 4 tablespoons cocoa powder
- 1 teaspoon vanilla extract
- 1 cup mint, chopped
- 2 cups coconut cream
- 4 tablespoons stevia

Directions:

- In your food processor, combine the coconut oil with the cocoa powder, the cream, and the other ingredients, pulse well, divide into bowls and serve cold.

Nutrition:

- Calories 514, Fat 56, Fiber 3.9, Carbs 7.8, Protein 3

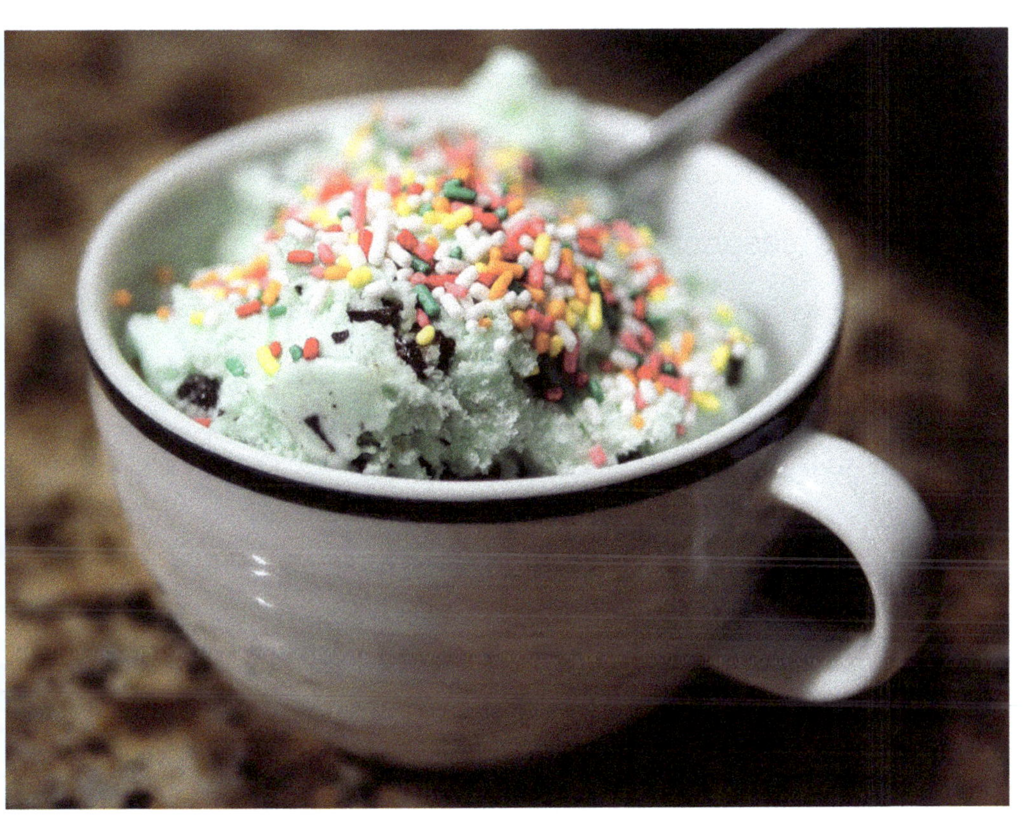

# Cranberries Cake

• Preparation Time: 10 minutes | Cooking Time: 30 minutes | Servings: 6

Ingredients:

- 2 cups coconut flour
- 2 tablespoon coconut oil, melted
- 3 tablespoons stevia
- 1 tablespoon cocoa powder, unsweetened
- 2 tablespoons flaxseed mixed with 3

tablespoons water

- 1 cup cranberries
- 1 cup coconut cream
- ¼ teaspoon vanilla extract
- ½ teaspoon baking powder

Directions:

• In a bowl, combine the coconut flour with the coconut oil, the stevia, and the other ingredients, and whisk well.

- Pour this into a cake pan lined with parchment paper, introduce it to the oven and cook at 360 degrees F for 30 minutes.
- Cool down, slice, and serve.

Nutrition:

- Calories 244, Fat 16.7, Fiber 11.8, Carbs 21.3, Protein 4.4

# Sweet Zucchini Buns

• Preparation Time: 10 minutes | Cooking Time: 30 minutes | Servings: 8

Ingredients:

- 1 cup almond flour
- 1/3 cup coconut flesh, unsweetened and shredded
- 1 cup zucchinis, grated
- 2 tablespoons stevia
- 1 teaspoon baking soda
- ½ teaspoon cinnamon powder
- 3 tablespoons flaxseed mixed with 4 tablespoons water
- 1 cup coconut cream

Directions:

• In a bowl, mix the almond flour with the coconut flesh, the zucchinis, and the other ingredients, stir well until you obtain a dough, shape 8 buns, and arrange them on a baking sheet lined with parchment paper.

- Introduce it in the oven at 350 degrees and bake for 30 minutes.
- Serve these sweet buns warm.

Nutrition:

- Calories 169, Fat 15.3, Fiber 3.9, Carbs 6.4, Protein 3.2

# Lime Custard

• Preparation Time: 10 minutes | Cooking Time: 20 minutes | Servings: 6

Ingredients:

• pint almond milk

• 4 tablespoons lime zest, grated

• 3 tablespoons lime juice

• 3 tablespoons flaxseed mixed with 4 tablespoons water

• tablespoons stevia

• 2 teaspoons vanilla extract

Directions:

• In a bowl, combine the almond milk with the lime zest, lime juice, and the other ingredients, whisk well and divide into 4 ramekins.

• Bake in the oven at 360 degrees F for 30 minutes.

• Cool the custard down and serve.

Nutrition:

- Calories 234, Fat 21.6, Fiber 4.3, Carbs 9, Protein 3.5

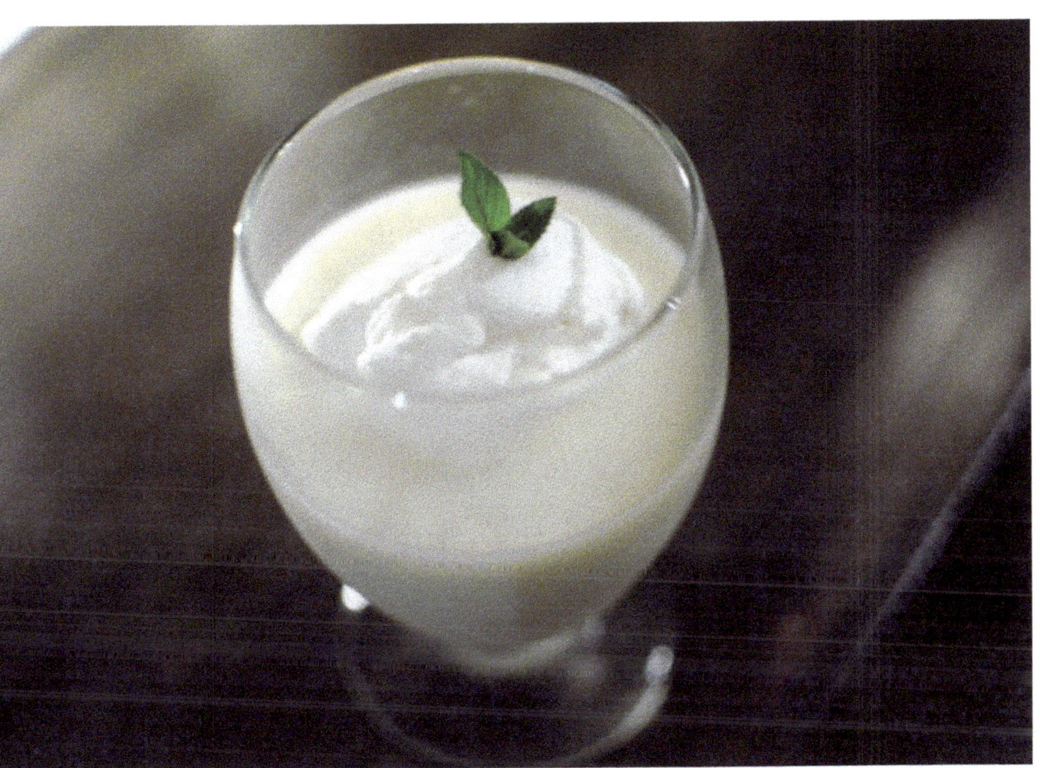

# Chocolate Fudge

Preparation Time: 10 minutes | Cooking Time: 0 minute | Servings: 12

Ingredients:

- 4 oz unsweetened dark chocolate
- 3/4 cup coconut butter
- 15 drops liquid stevia
- 1 tsp vanilla extract

Directions:

- Melt coconut butter and dark chocolate.
- Add ingredients to the large bowl and combine well.
- Pour mixture into a silicone loaf pan and place in the refrigerator until set.
- Cut into pieces and serve.

Nutrition:

- Calories: 283 Total Carbohydrate: 10 g

Cholesterol: 3 mg Total Fat: 8 g Fiber: 2 g

Protein: 9 g Sodium: 271 mg

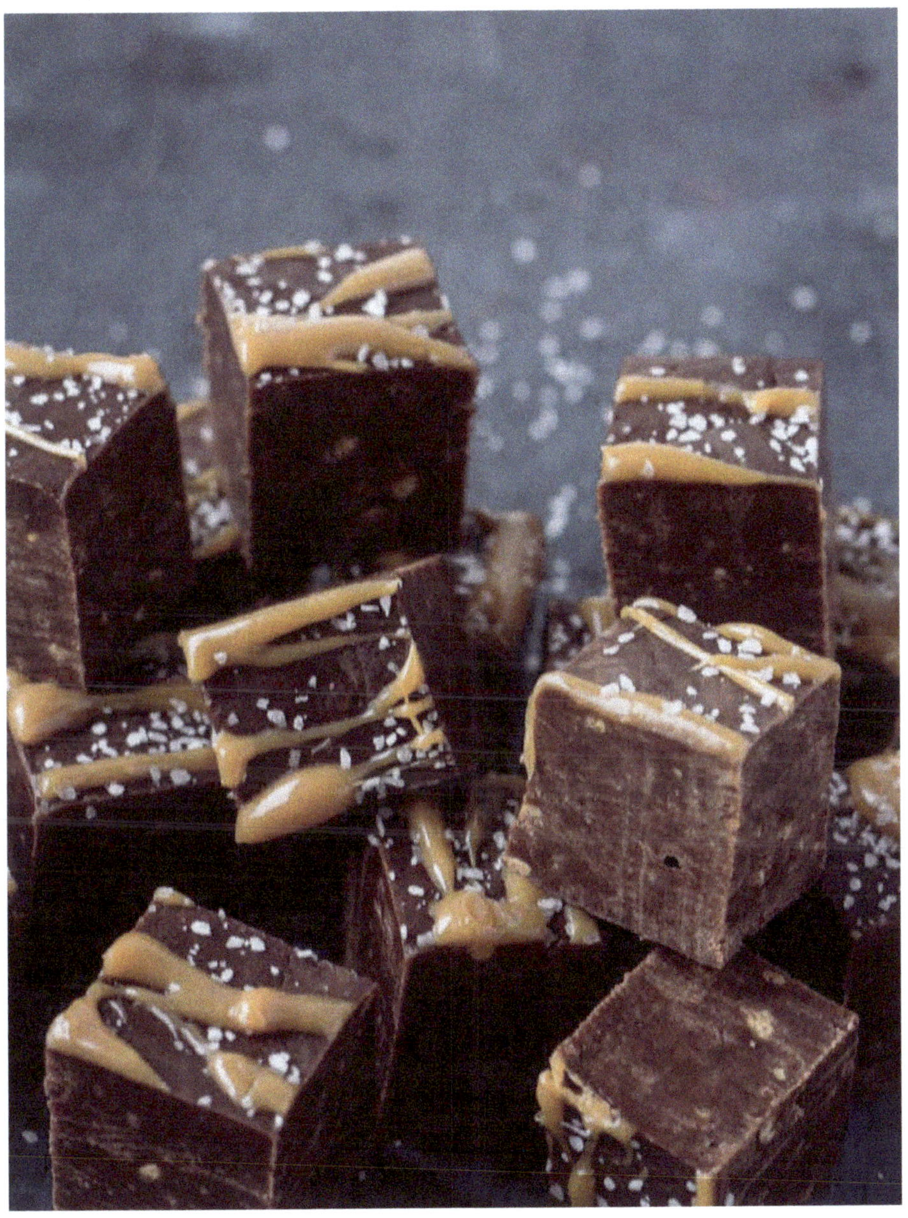

# Chocó Chia Pudding

Preparation Time: 10 minutes | Cooking Time: 0 minutes | Servings:  6

Ingredients:

- 2 1/2 cups coconut milk
- 2 scoops stevia extract powder
- 6 tbsp cocoa powder
- 1/2 cup chia seeds
- 1/2 tsp vanilla extract
- 1/8 cup xylitol
- 1/8 tsp salt

Directions:

- Add all ingredients into the blender and blend until smooth.
- Pour mixture into the glass container and place in the refrigerator.
- Serve chilled and enjoy.

Nutrition: Calories: 178 Total Carbohydrate: 3 g

Cholesterol: 3 mg Total Fat: 17 g Fiber: g

Protein: 9 g Sodium: 297 mg

# Raspberry Chia Pudding

• Preparation Time: 3 hours 10 minutes | Cooking Time: 0 minute | Servings: 2

Ingredients:

- 4 tbsp chia seeds
- 1 cup of coconut milk
- 1/2 cup raspberries

Directions:

• Add raspberry and coconut milk in a blender and blend until smooth.

• Pour mixture into the Mason jar.

• Add chia seeds in a jar and stir well.

• Close the jar tightly with the lid and shake well.

• Place in the refrigerator for 3 hours.

• Serve chilled and enjoy.

Nutrition:

- Calories: 189 Total Carbohydrate: 6 g

Cholesterol: 3 mg Total Fat: 7 g Fiber: 4 g

Protein: 12 g Sodium: 293 mg

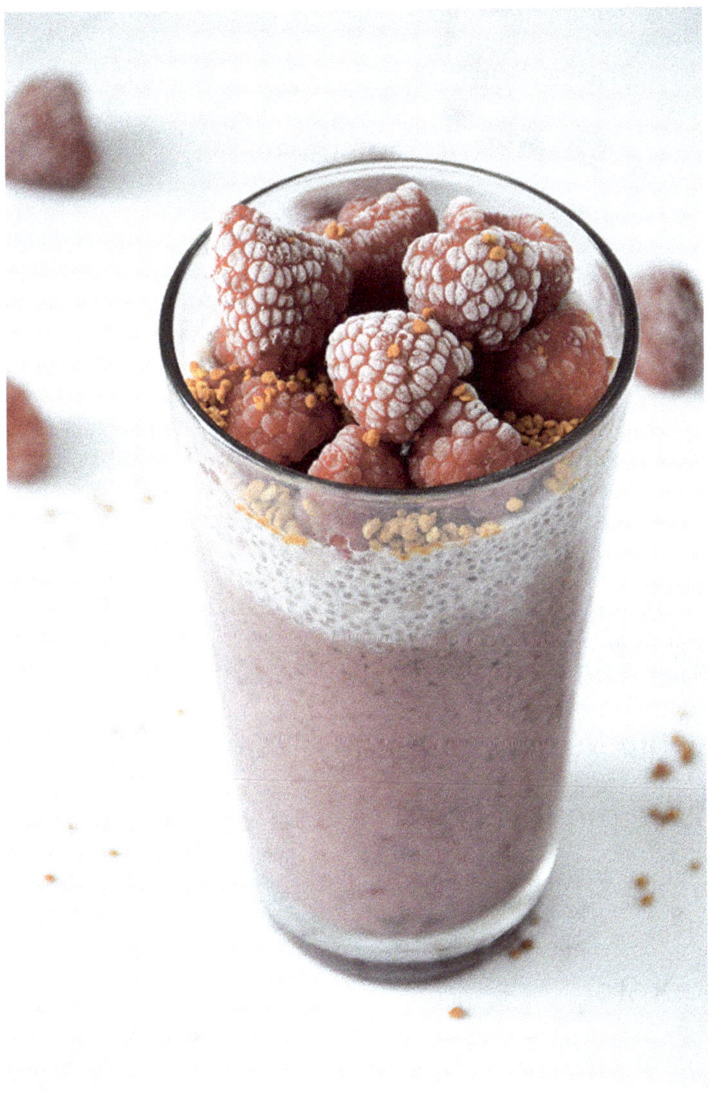

# Lemon Mousse

Preparation Time: 10 minutes | Cooking Time: 0 minute | Servings: 2

Ingredients:

- 14 oz coconut milk
- 12 drops liquid stevia
- 1/2 tsp lemon extract
- 1/4 tsp turmeric

Directions:

• Place coconut milk in the refrigerator overnight. Scoop out thick cream into a mixing bowl. • Add remaining ingredients to the bowl and whip using a hand mixer until smooth. • Transfer mousse mixture to a zip-lock bag and pipe into small serving glasses. Place in the

refrigerator.

• Serve chilled and enjoy.

Nutrition:

- Calories: 189 Total Carbohydrate: 2 g

Cholesterol: 13 mg Total Fat: 7 g Fiber: 2 g

Protein: 15 g Sodium: 321 mg

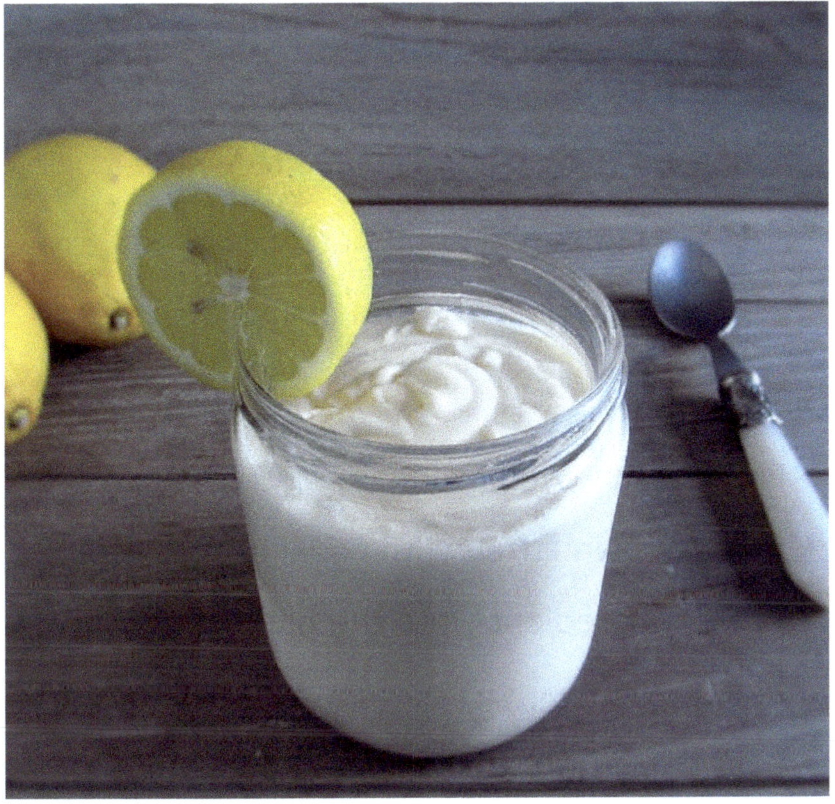

# Almond Butter Brownies

• Preparation Time: 10 minutes | Cooking Time: 20 minutes | Servings: 4

Ingredients:

- 1 scoop protein powder
- 2 tbsp cocoa powder
- 1/2 cup almond butter, melted
- 1 cup bananas, overripe

Directions:

• Preheat the oven to 350 F/ 176 C.

• Spray brownie tray with cooking spray.

• Add all ingredients into the blender and blend until smooth.

• Pour batter into the prepared dish and bake in a preheated oven for 20 minutes. • Serve and enjoy.

Nutrition:

- Calories: 214 Total Carbohydrate: 2 g

Cholesterol: 73 mg Total Fat: 7 g Fiber: 2g

Protein: 19 g Sodium: 308 g

# Coconut Peanut Butter Fudge

• Preparation Time: 1 hour 15 minutes | Cooking Time: 0 minute | Servings: 20

Ingredients:

- 12 oz smooth peanut butter
- 3 tbsp coconut oil
- 4 tbsp coconut cream
- 15 drops liquid stevia
- Pinch of salt

Directions:

• Line a baking tray with parchment paper.

• Melt coconut oil in a saucepan over low heat.

• Add peanut butter, coconut cream, stevia, and salt in a saucepan. Stir well. • Pour fudge mixture into the prepared baking tray and place in the refrigerator for 1 hour. • Cut into pieces and serve.

Nutrition:

• Calories: 189 Total Carbohydrate: 2 g Cholesterol: 13 mg Total Fat: 7 g Fiber: 2 g Protein: 10 g Sodium: 301 mg

# Simple Almond Butter Fudge

Preparation Time: 15 minutes | Cooking Time: 0 minutes | Servings: 8

Ingredients:

- 1/2 cup almond butter
- 15 drops liquid stevia
- 2 1/2 tbsp coconut oil

Directions:

• Combine almond butter and coconut oil in a saucepan. Gently warm until melted. • Add stevia and stir well.

• Pour mixture into the candy container and place in the refrigerator until set. • Serve and enjoy.

Nutrition:

• Calories: 198 Total Carbohydrate: 5 g

Cholesterol: 12 mg Total Fat: 10 g Fiber: 2 g

Protein: 6 g Sodium: 257 mg

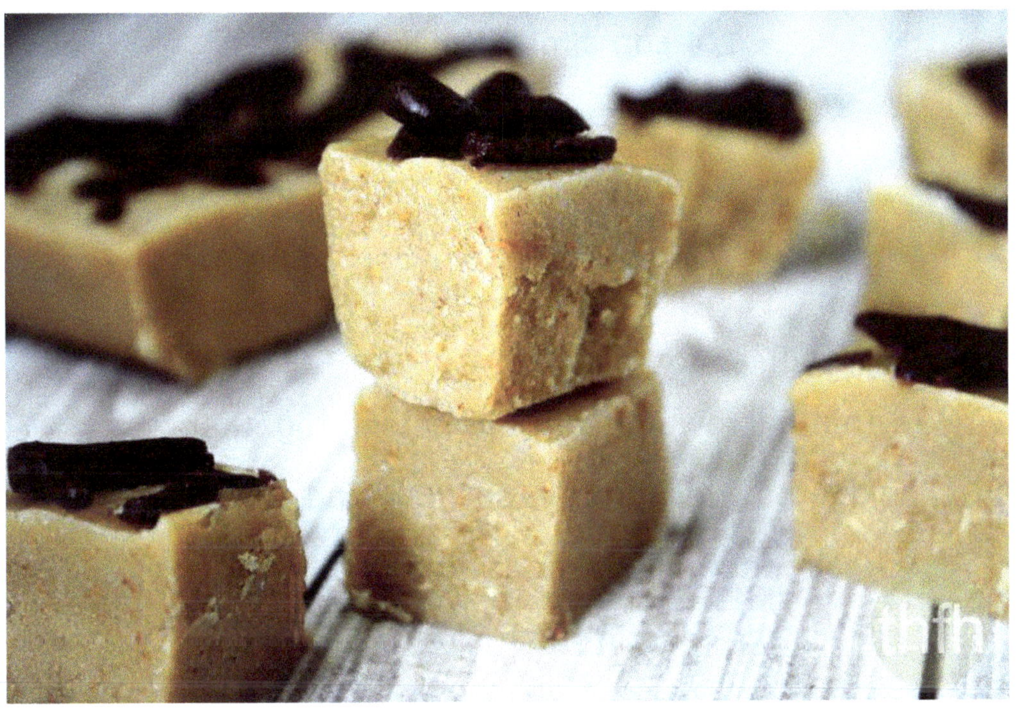

# Quick Chocó Brownie

Preparation Time: 10 minutes | Cooking Time: 2 minutes | Servings: 1

Ingredients:

- 1/4 cup almond milk
- 1 tbsp cocoa powder
- 1 scoop chocolate protein powder
- 1/2 tsp baking powder

Directions:

- In a microwave-safe mug blend together baking powder, protein powder, and cocoa. • Add almond milk to the mug and stir well.
- Place the mug in the microwave and microwave for 30 seconds.
- Serve and enjoy.

Nutrition:

- Calories: 231 Total Carbohydrate: 2 g

Cholesterol: 13 mg Total Fat: 15 g Fiber: 2 g

Protein: 8 g Sodium: 298 mg

# Avocado Pudding

Preparation Time: 10 minutes | Cooking Time: 0 minute | Servings: 8

Ingredients:

* 2 ripe avocados, peeled, pitted, and cut into pieces
* 1 tbsp fresh lime juice
* 14 oz can coconut milk
* 80 drops of liquid stevia
* 2 tsp vanilla extract

Directions:

* Add all ingredients into the blender and blend until smooth.
* Serve and enjoy.

Nutrition:

* Calories: 209 Total Carbohydrate: 6 g
Cholesterol: 13 mg Total Fat: 7 g Fiber: 2 g
Protein: 17 g Sodium: 193 mg

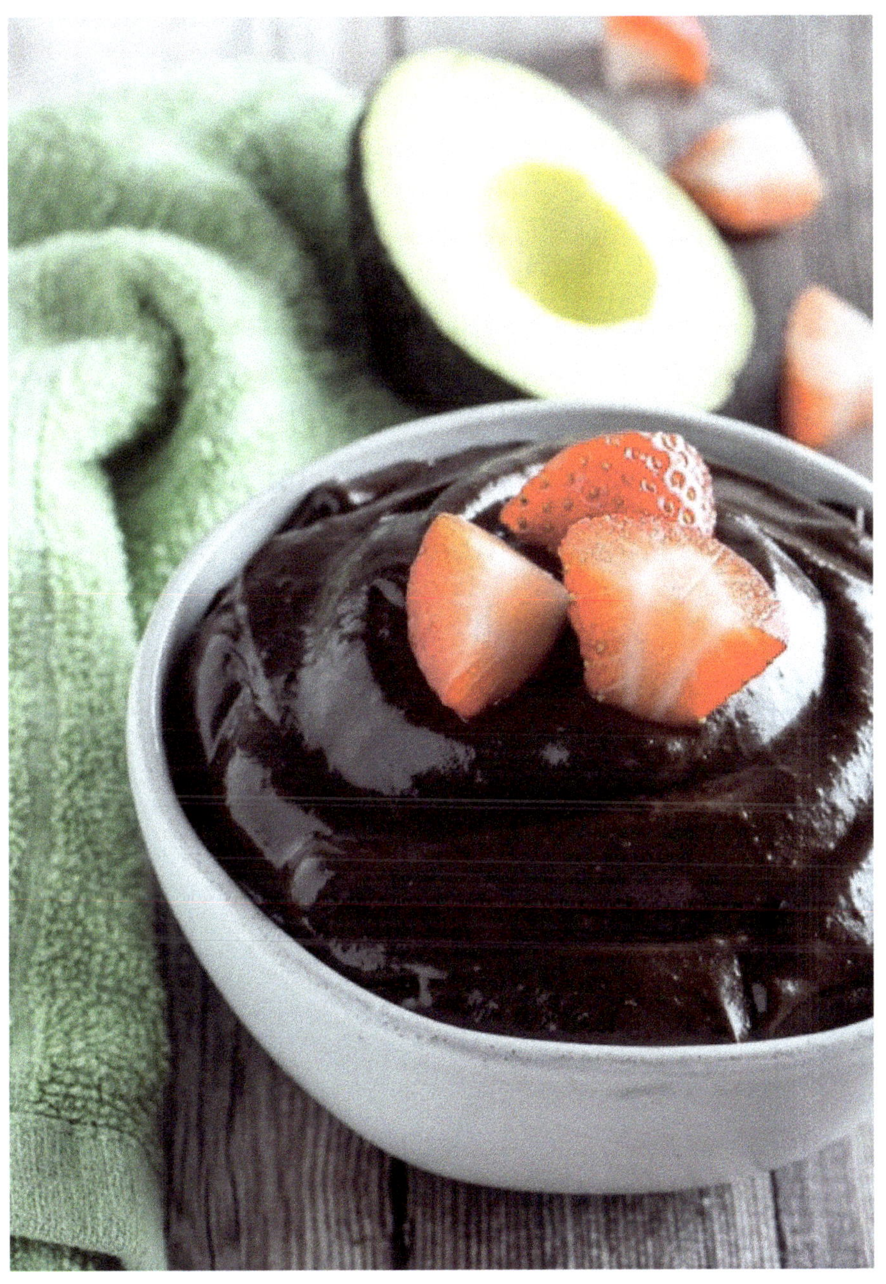

# Walnut & Chocolate Bars

• Preparation Time: 15-30 minutes | Cooking Time: 60 minutes | Servings: 4

Ingredients:

- 1 cup walnuts
- 3 tbsp sunflower seeds
- 2 tbsp unsweetened chocolate chips
- 1 tbsp unsweetened cocoa powder
- 1 ½ tsp vanilla extract
- ¼ tsp cinnamon powder
- 2 tbsp melted coconut oil
- 2 tbsp toasted almond meal
- 2 tsp pure maple syrup

Directions:

• In a food processor, add the walnuts, sunflower seeds, chocolate chips, cocoa powder, vanilla extract, cinnamon powder, coconut oil, almond meal, maple syrup, and blitz a few times until coarsely combined.

- Line a flat baking sheet with plastic wrap, pour the mixture onto the sheet and place another plastic wrap on top. Use a rolling pin to flatten the mixture and then remove the top plastic wrap.
- Freeze the snack until firm, 1 hour.
- Remove from the freezer, cut into 1 ½-inch bars and enjoy immediately.

Nutrition:

- Calories 302 Fats 23. 9g Carbs 20. 2g Protein 5. 2g

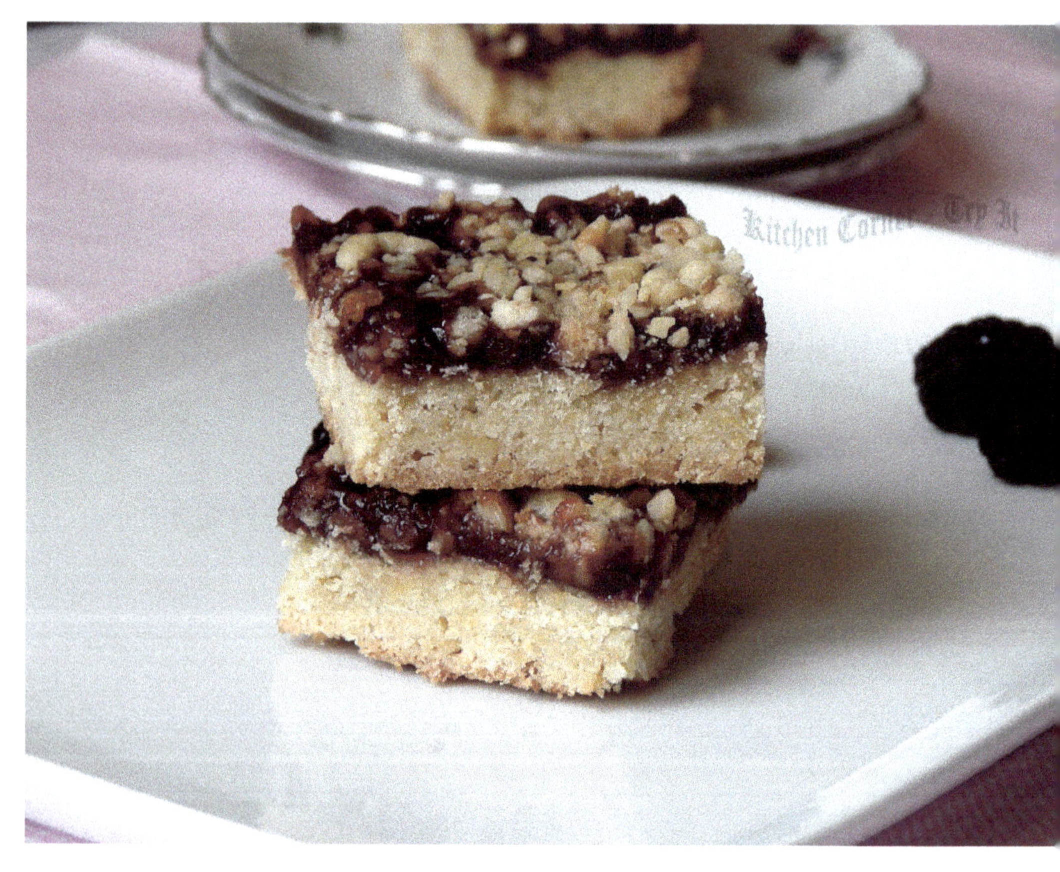

# Nectarine Chia Pudding

- Preparation Time: 5-15 minutes | Cooking Time: 5 minutes + 4 hour refrigeration | Servings: 4

Ingredients:

- 1 cup of coconut milk
- ½ tsp vanilla extract
- 3 tbsp chia seeds
- ½ cup granola
- 2/3 cup chopped sweet nectarine

Directions:

- In a medium bowl, mix the coconut milk, vanilla, and chia seeds until well combined. • Divide the mixture between 4 breakfast cups and refrigerate for at least 4 hours to allow the mixture to gel.
- After, top with the granola and nectarine.

Enjoy immediately.

Nutrition:

- Calories 72 Fats 3. 4g Carbs 7. 8g Protein 2. 6g

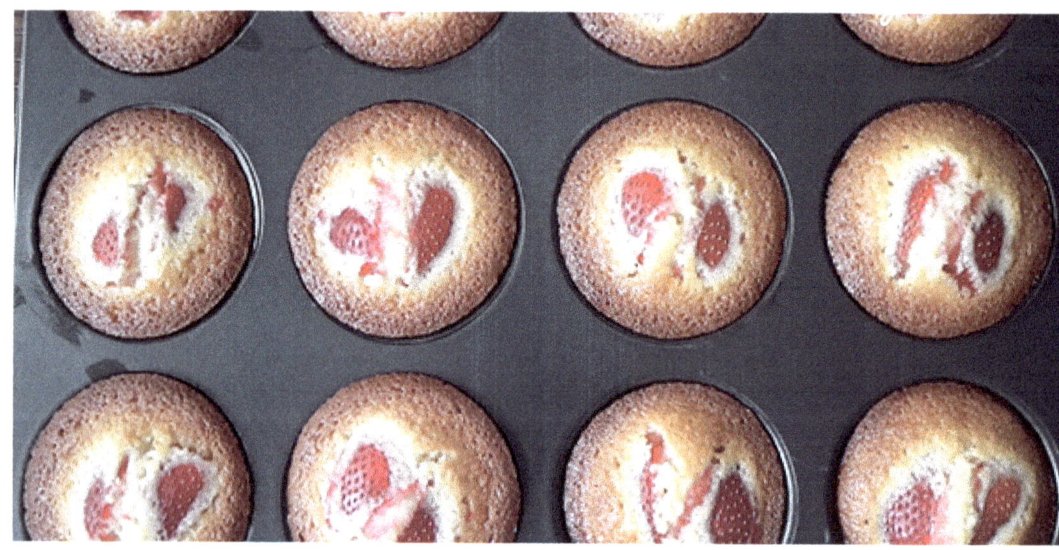

# Energizing Cinnamon Detox Tonic

• Preparation Time: 15-30 minutes | Cooking Time: 15 minutes | Servings: 2

Ingredients:

- 4 sticks of cinnamon 2 inches each
- 1 small lemon slice
- 1/8 teaspoon of cayenne pepper
- 1/8 teaspoon of ground turmeric
- 1 teaspoon of maple syrup
- 1 teaspoon of apple cider vinegar
- 2 cups of boiling water

Directions:

- Pour the boiling water into a small saucepan, add and stir the cinnamon sticks, then let it rest for 8 to 10 minutes, before covering the pan.

- Pass the mixture through a strainer and into the liquid, add the cayenne pepper, turmeric, cinnamon and stir properly.

- Add the maple syrup, vinegar, and lemon slice.

- Add and stir an infused lemon and serve immediately.

Nutrition:

- Calories:80 Cal, Carbohydrates:0g, Protein:0g, Fats:0g, Fiber:0g.

- Cinnamon Cherry Cider | Servings: 16

- Preparation Time: 15-30 minutes | Cooking Time: 4 hours and 5 minutes

Ingredients:

- 2 cinnamon sticks, each about 3 inches long

- 6-ounce of cherry gelatin

- 4 quarts of apple cider

Directions:

- Using a 6-quarts slow cooker, pour the apple cider and add the cinnamon stick. • Stir, then cover the slow cooker with its lid. Plug the cooker and let it cook for 3 hours at the

high heat setting or until it is heated thoroughly.

- Then add and stir the gelatin properly, then continue cooking for another hour. • When done, remove the cinnamon sticks and serve the drink hot or cold.

Nutrition:

- Calories:100 Cal, Carbohydrates:0g, Protein:0g, Fats:0g, Fiber:0g.

# Warm Pomegranate Punch

• Preparation Time: 15-30 minutes | Cooking

Time: 2 hours and 15 minutes | Servings: 10

Ingredients:

- 3 cinnamon sticks, each about 3 inches long
- 12 whole cloves
- 1/2 cup of coconut sugar
- 1/3 cup of lemon juice
- 32 fluid ounce of pomegranate juice
- 32 fluid ounce of apple juice, unsweetened
- 16 fluid ounce of brewed tea

Directions:

• Using a 4-quart slow cooker, pour the lemon juice, pomegranate, juice apple juice, tea, and then sugar.

• Wrap the whole cloves and cinnamon stick in a cheesecloth, tie its corners with a string, and immerse it in the liquid present in the slow cooker.

• Then cover it with the lid, plug in the slow cooker and let it cook at the low heat setting for 3 hours or until it is heated thoroughly.

• When done, discard the cheesecloth bag and serve it hot or cold.

Nutrition:

• Calories:253 Cal, Carbohydrates:58g, Protein:7g, Fats:2g, Fiber:3g.

# Rich Truffle Hot Chocolate

• Preparation Time: 15-30 minutes | Cooking Time: 1 hour and 10 minutes | Servings: 4

Ingredients:

• 1/3 cup of cocoa powder, unsweetened

• 1/3 cup of coconut sugar

• 1/8 teaspoon of salt

• 1/8 teaspoon of ground cinnamon

• 1 teaspoon of vanilla extract, unsweetened

• 32 fluid ounce of coconut milk

Directions:

• Using a 2 quarts slow cooker, add all the ingredients, and stir properly.

• Cover it with the lid, then plug in the slow cooker and cook it for 2 hours on the high heat setting or until it is heated thoroughly.

• When done, serve right away.

Nutrition:

• Calories:67 Cal, Carbohydrates:13g,

Protein:2g, Fats:2g, Fiber:2. 3g.

# Warm Spiced Lemon Drink

• Preparation Time: 15-30 minutes | Cooking Time: 2 hours and 10 minutes | Servings: 12

Ingredients:

- 1 cinnamon stick, about 3 inches long
- 1/2 teaspoon of whole cloves
- 2 cups of coconut sugar
- 4 fluid of ounce pineapple juice
- 1/2 cup and 2 tablespoons of lemon juice
- 12 fluid ounce of orange juice
- 2 1/2 quarts of water

Directions:

• Pour water into a 6-quarts slow cooker and stir the sugar and lemon juice properly. • Wrap the cinnamon, the whole cloves in cheesecloth, and tie its corners with string. • Immerse this cheesecloth bag in the liquid present in the slow cooker and cover it with the lid.

• Then plug in the slow cooker and let it cook on a high heat setting for 2 hours or until it is heated thoroughly.

• When done, discard the cheesecloth bag and serve the drink hot or cold.

Nutrition:

• Calories:15 Cal, Carbohydrates:3. 2g, Protein:0. 1g, Fats:0g,  Fiber:0g.

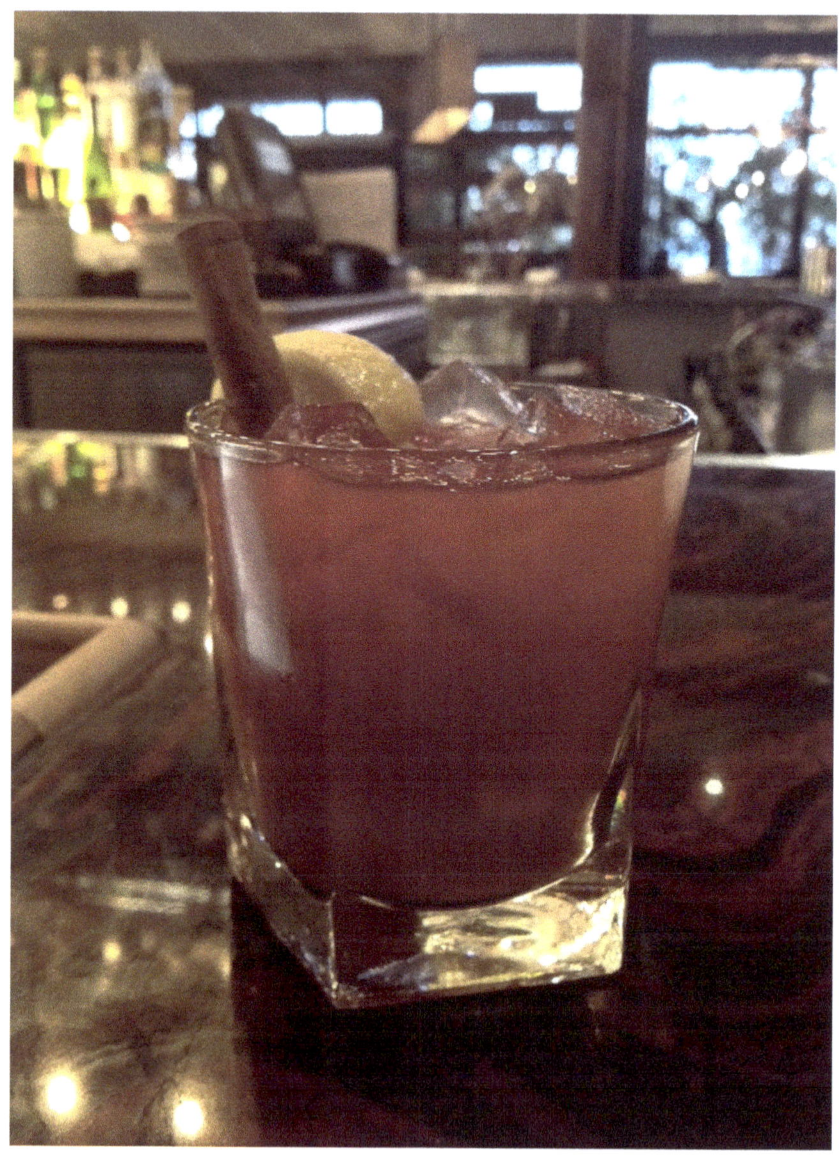

# Ultimate Mulled Wine

• Preparation Time: 15-30 minutes | Cooking Time: 35 minutes | Servings: 6

Ingredients:

- 1 cup of cranberries, fresh
- 2 oranges, juiced
- 1 tablespoon of whole cloves
- 2 cinnamon sticks, each about 3 inches long
- 1 tablespoon of star anise
- 1/3 cup of honey
- 8 fluid ounce of apple cider
- 8 fluid ounce of cranberry juice
- 24 fluid ounce of red wine

Directions:

• Using a 4 quarts slow cooker, add all the ingredients, and stir properly.

• Cover it with the lid, then plug in the slow

cooker and cook it for 30 minutes on the high heat

setting or until it gets warm thoroughly.

• When done, strain the wine and serve right away.

Nutrition:

• Calories:202 Cal, Carbohydrates:25g, Protein:0g, Fats:0g, Fiber:0g.

# Pleasant Lemonade

- Preparation Time: 15-30 minutes | Cooking Time: 3 hours and 15 minutes | Servings: 10 servings

Ingredients:

- Cinnamon sticks for serving
- 2 cups of coconut sugar
- 1/4 cup of honey
- 3 cups of lemon juice. fresh
- 32 fluid ounce of water

Directions:

- Using a 4-quarts slow cooker, place all the ingredients except for the cinnamon sticks and stir properly.
- Cover it with the lid, then plug in the slow cooker and cook it for 3 hours on the low heat setting or until it is heated thoroughly.

• When done, stir properly and serve with the cinnamon sticks.

Nutrition:

• Calories:146 Cal, Carbohydrates:34g, Protein:0g, Fats:0g, Fiber:0g.

# Pumpkin Spice Frappuccino

Preparation Time: 5 minutes | Cooking Time: 0 minute | Servings: 2

Ingredients:

- ½ teaspoon ground ginger

- 1/8 teaspoon allspice

- ½ teaspoon ground cinnamon

- 2 tablespoons coconut sugar

- 1/8 teaspoon nutmeg

- ¼ teaspoon ground cloves

- 1 teaspoon vanilla extract, unsweetened

- 2 teaspoons instant coffee

- 2 cups almond milk, unsweetened

- 1 cup of ice cubes

Directions:

• Place all the ingredients in the order in a food processor or blender and then pulse for 2 to 3 minutes at high speed until smooth.

 • Pour the Frappuccino into two glasses and then serve.

Nutrition:

 • Calories: 490 Fat: 9g Protein: 12g Sugar: 11g

# Cookie Dough Milkshake

Preparation Time: 5 minutes | Cooking Time: 0 minute | Servings: 2

Ingredients:

- 2 tablespoons cookie dough

- 5 dates, pitted

- 2 teaspoons chocolate chips

- 1/2 teaspoon vanilla extract, unsweetened

- 1/2 cup almond milk, unsweetened

- 1 ½ cup almond milk ice cubes

Directions:

• Place all the ingredients in the order in a food processor or blender and then pulse for 2 to 3 minutes at high speed until smooth.

• Pour the milkshake into two glasses and then serve with some cookie dough balls.

Nutrition:

- Calories: 240 Fat: 13g Protein: 21g Sugar: 9g

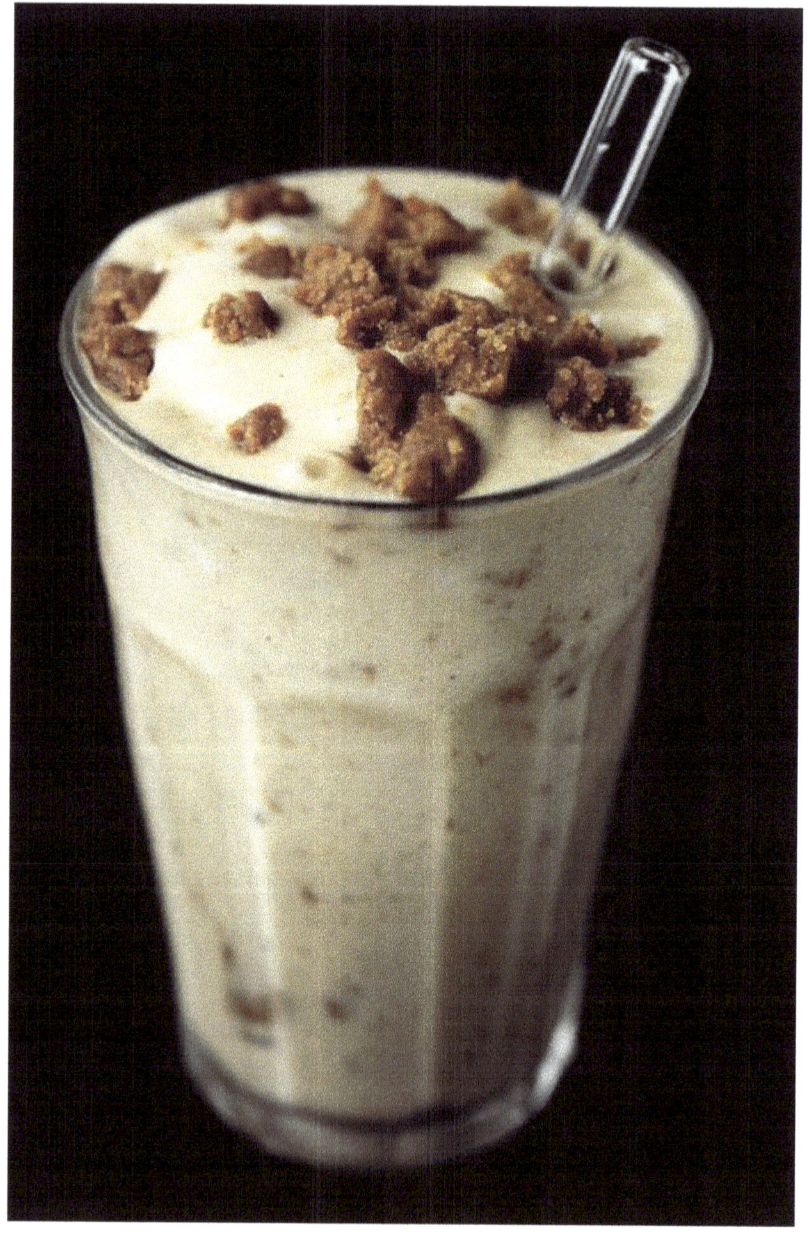

# Strawberry and Hemp Smoothie

Preparation Time: 5 minutes | Cooking Time: 0 minute  | Servings: 2

Ingredients:

- 3 cups fresh strawberries
- 2 tablespoons hemp seeds
- 1/2 teaspoon vanilla extract, unsweetened
- 1/8 teaspoon sea salt
- 2 tablespoons maple syrup
- 1 cup vegan yogurt
- 1 cup almond milk, unsweetened
- 1 cup of ice cubes
- 2 tablespoons hemp protein

Directions:

• Place all the ingredients in the order in a food processor or blender, except for protein powder, and then pulse for 2 to 3 minutes at high speed until smooth.

• Pour the smoothie into two glasses and then serve.

Nutrition:

• Calories: 510 Fat: 18g Protein: 26g Sugar: 12g

# Blueberry, Hazelnut, and Hemp Smoothie

Preparation Time: 5 minutes | Cooking Time: 0 minute | Servings: 2

Ingredients:

- 2 tablespoons hemp seeds
- 1 ½ cups frozen blueberries
- 2 tablespoons chocolate protein powder
- 1/2 teaspoon vanilla extract, unsweetened
- 2 tablespoons chocolate hazelnut butter
- 1 small frozen banana
- 3/4 cup almond milk

Directions:

- Place all the ingredients in the order in a food processor or blender and then pulse for 2 to 3 minutes at high speed until smooth.

- Pour the smoothie into two glasses and then serve.

Nutrition:

- Calories: 195 Fat: 14g Protein: 36g Sugar: 10g

# Mango Lassi

Preparation Time: 5 minutes | Cooking Time: 0 minute | Servings: 2

Ingredients:

- 1 ¼ cup mango pulp
- 1 tablespoon coconut sugar
- 1/8 teaspoon salt
- 1/2 teaspoon lemon juice
- 1/4 cup almond milk, unsweetened
- 1/4 cup chilled water
- 1 cup cashew yogurt

Directions:

- Place all the ingredients in the order in a food processor or blender and then pulse for 2 to 3 minutes at high speed until smooth.
- Pour the lassi into two glasses and then serve.

Nutrition:

- Calories: 420 Fat: 12g Protein: 23g Sugar: 13g

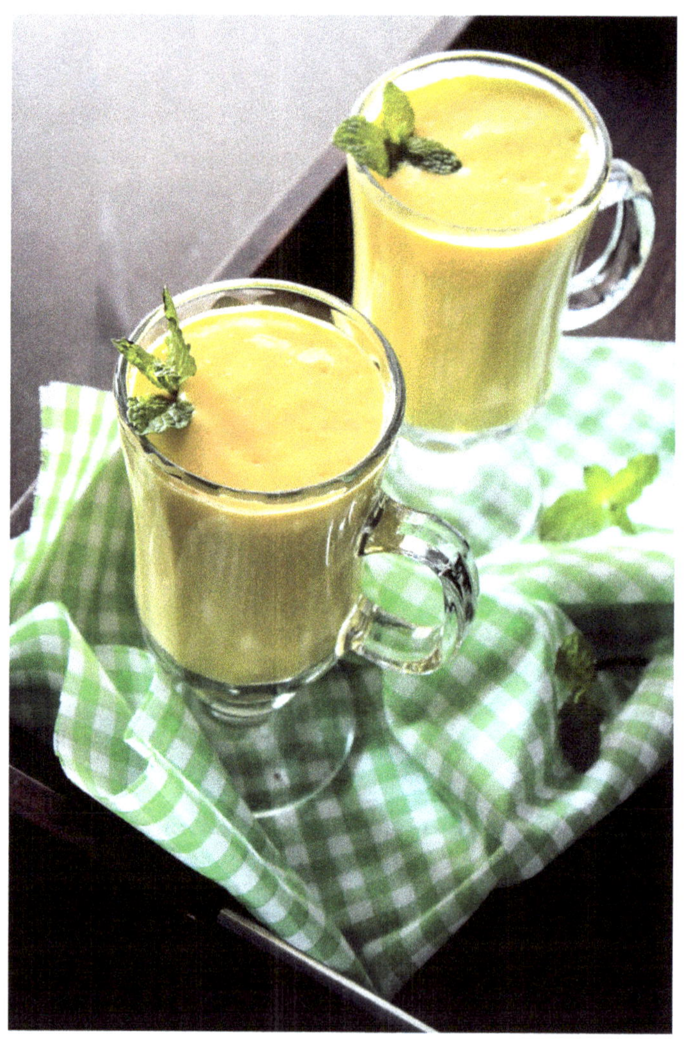

# Mocha Chocolate Shake

Preparation Time: 5 minutes | Cooking Time: 0 minute | Servings: 2

Ingredients:

- 1/4 cup hemp seeds
- 2 teaspoons cocoa powder, unsweetened
- 1/2 cup dates, pitted
- 1 tablespoon instant coffee powder
- 2 tablespoons flax seeds
- 2 1/2 cups almond milk, unsweetened
- 1/2 cup crushed ice

Directions:

• Place all the ingredients in the order in a food processor or blender and then pulse for 2 to 3 minutes at high speed until smooth.

• Pour the smoothie into two glasses and then serve.

Nutrition:

- Calories: 432 Fat: 18g Protein: 14g Sugar: 12g

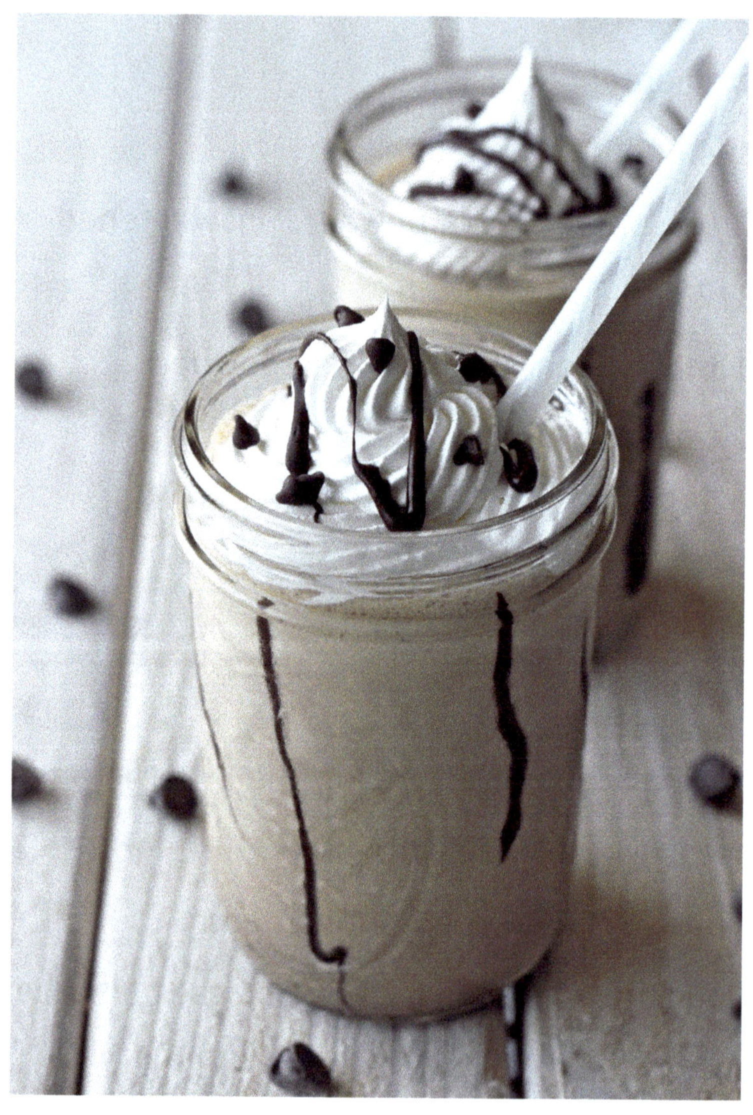

# Chard, Lettuce, and Ginger Smoothie

Preparation Time: 5 minutes | Cooking Time: 0 minute | Servings: 2

Ingredients:

- 10 Chard leaves, chopped

- inch piece of ginger, chopped

- 10 lettuce leaves, chopped

- ½ teaspoon black salt

- 2 pear, chopped

- 2 teaspoons coconut sugar

- ¼ teaspoon ground black pepper

- ¼ teaspoon salt

- 2 tablespoons lemon juice

- 2 cups of water

Directions:

• Place all the ingredients in the order in a food processor or blender and then pulse for 2 to 3 minutes at high speed until smooth.

 • Pour the smoothie into two glasses and then serve.

Nutrition:

 • Calories: 240 Fat: 4g Protein: 16g Sugar: 3g

# Red Beet, Pear, and Apple Smoothie

Preparation Time: 5 minutes | Cooking Time: 0 minute | Servings: 2

Ingredients:

- 1/2 of medium beet, peeled, chopped
- 1 tablespoon chopped cilantro
- 1 orange, juiced
- 1 medium pear, chopped
- 1 medium apple, cored, chopped
- 1/4 teaspoon ground black pepper
- 1/8 teaspoon rock salt
- 1 teaspoon coconut sugar
- 1/4 teaspoons salt
- 1 cup of water

Directions:

• Place all the ingredients in the order in a food processor or blender and then pulse for 2 to 3 minutes at high speed until smooth.

• Pour the smoothie into two glasses and then serve.

Nutrition:

• Calories: 240 Fat: 4g Protein: 16g Sugar: 3g

# Berry and Yogurt Smoothie

Preparation Time: 5 minutes | Cooking Time: 0 minute | Servings: 2

Ingredients:

- 2 small bananas
- 3 cups frozen mixed berries
- 1 ½ cup cashew yogurt
- 1/2 teaspoon vanilla extract, unsweetened
- 1/2 cup almond milk, unsweetened

Directions:

• Place all the ingredients in the order in a food processor or blender and then pulse for 2 to 3 minutes at high speed until smooth.

• Pour the smoothie into two glasses and then serve.

Nutrition:

• Calories: 291 Fat: 9g Protein: 17g Sugar: 5g

# Chocolate and Cherry Smoothie

Preparation Time: 5 minutes | Cooking Time: 0 minute | Servings: 2

Ingredients:

- 4 cups frozen cherries

- 2 tablespoons cocoa powder

- 1 scoop of protein powder

- 1 teaspoon maple syrup

- 2 cups almond milk, unsweetened

Directions:

• Place all the ingredients in the order in a food processor or blender and then pulse for 2 to 3 minutes at high speed until smooth.

• Pour the smoothie into two glasses and then serve.

Nutrition:

- Calories: 247 Fat: 3g Protein: 18g Sugar: 3g

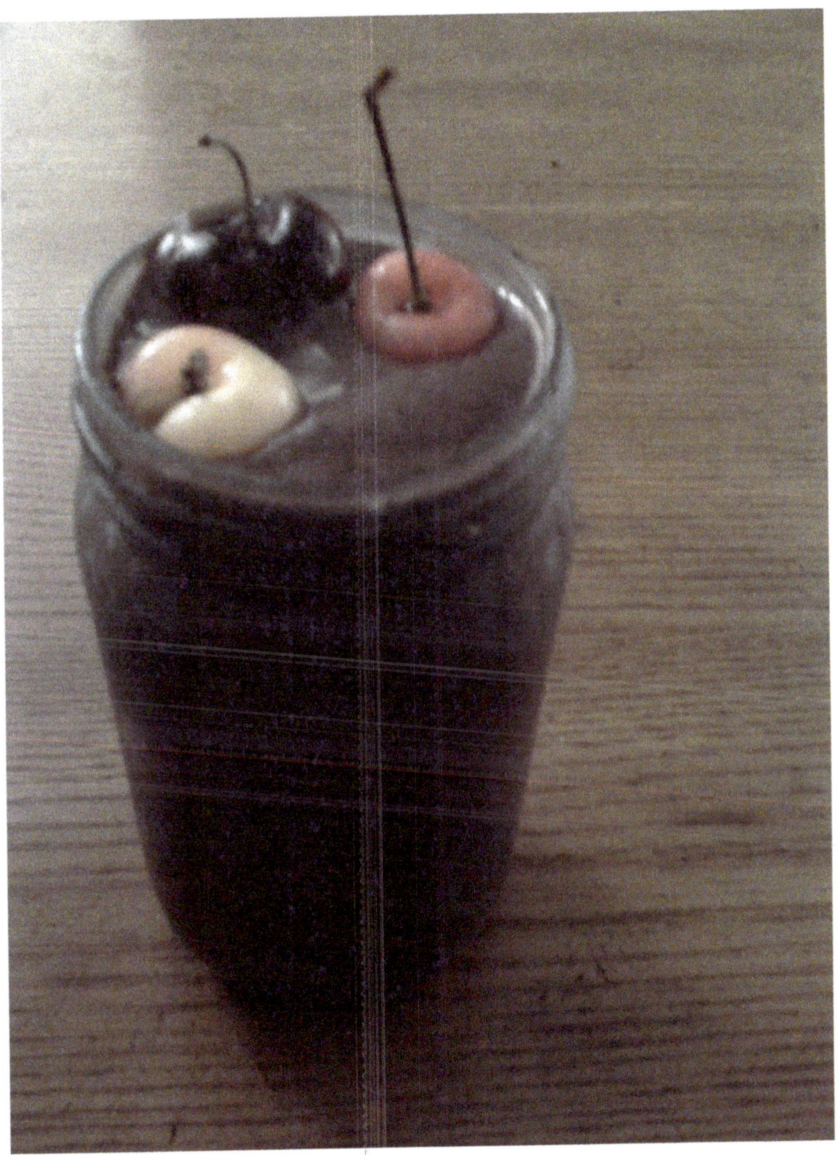

# Banana Weight Loss Juice

Preparation Time: 10 minutes | Cooking Time: 0 minutes | Servings: 1

Ingredients:

- Water (1/3 C.)

- Apple (1, Sliced)

- Orange (1, Sliced)

- Banana (1, Sliced)

- Lemon Juice (1 T.)

Directions:

• Simply place everything into your blender, blend on high for twenty seconds, and then pour into your glass.

Nutrition:

• Calories: 289 Total Carbohydrate: 2 g Cholesterol: 3 mg Total Fat: 17 g Fiber: 2 g Protein: 7 g Sodium: 163 mg

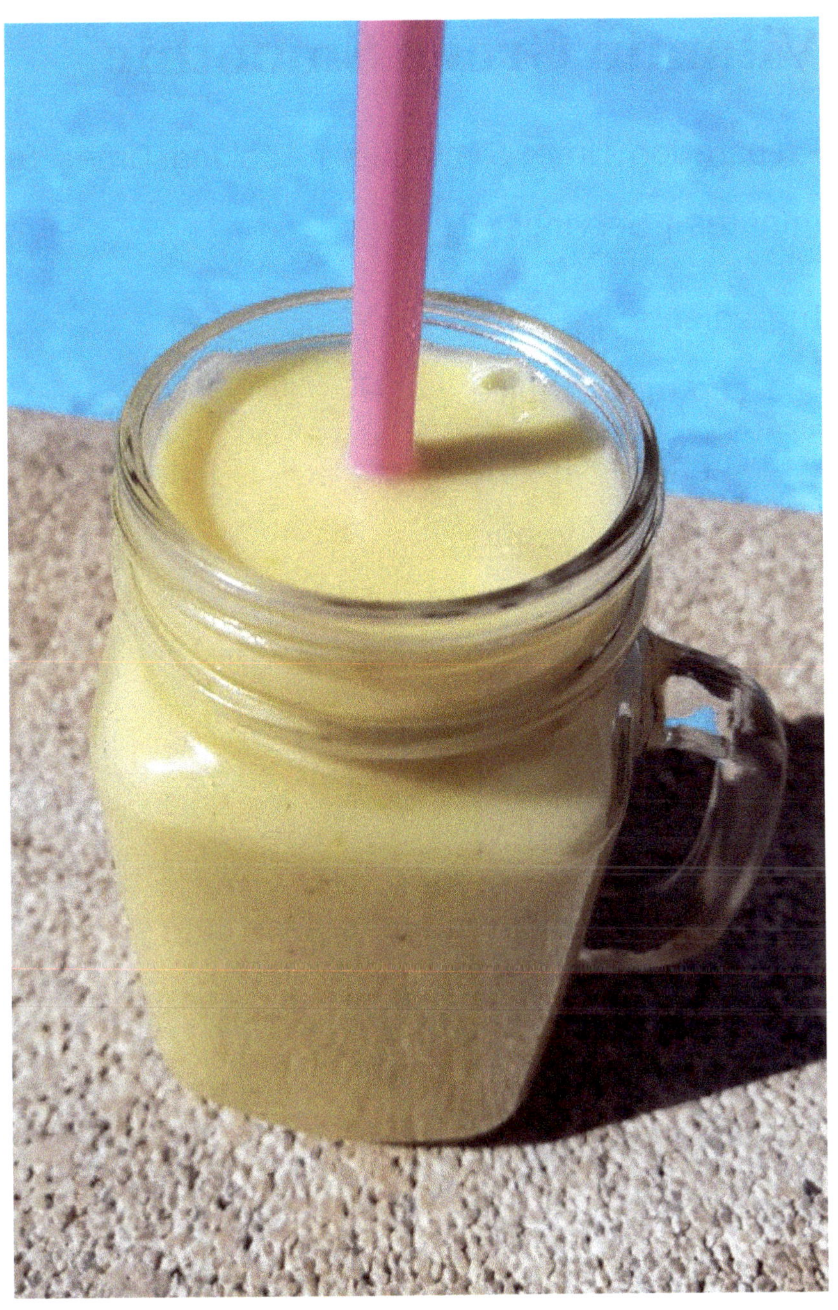

# Vitamin Green Smoothie

Preparation Time: 5 minutes | Cooking Time:  5 minutes | Servings: 2

Ingredients:

- 1 cup milk or juice
- 1 cup spinach or kale
- ½ cup plain yogurt
- 1 kiwi
- 1 Tbsp chia or flax
- 1 tsp vanilla

Directions:

- Mix the milk or juice and greens until smooth. Add the remaining ingredients and continue blending until smooth again.
- Enjoy your delicious drink!

Nutrition:

- Calories 397 Fat 36.4 g Carbohydrates 4 g Sugar 1 g Protein 14.7 g Cholesterol 4 mg

# Strawberry Grapefruit Smoothie

Preparation Time: 5 minutes | Cooking Time: 5 minutes | Servings: 2

Ingredients:

- 1 banana
- ½ cup strawberries, frozen
- 1 grapefruit
- ¼ cup milk
- ¼ cup plain yogurt
- 2 Tbsp honey
- ½ tsp ginger, chopped

Directions:

- Using a mixer, blend all the ingredients.
- When smooth, top your drink with a slice of grapefruit and enjoy it!

Nutrition:

- Calories 233 Fat 7.9 g Carbohydrates 3.2 g
Sugar 0.1 g Protein 35.6 g Cholesterol 32 mg

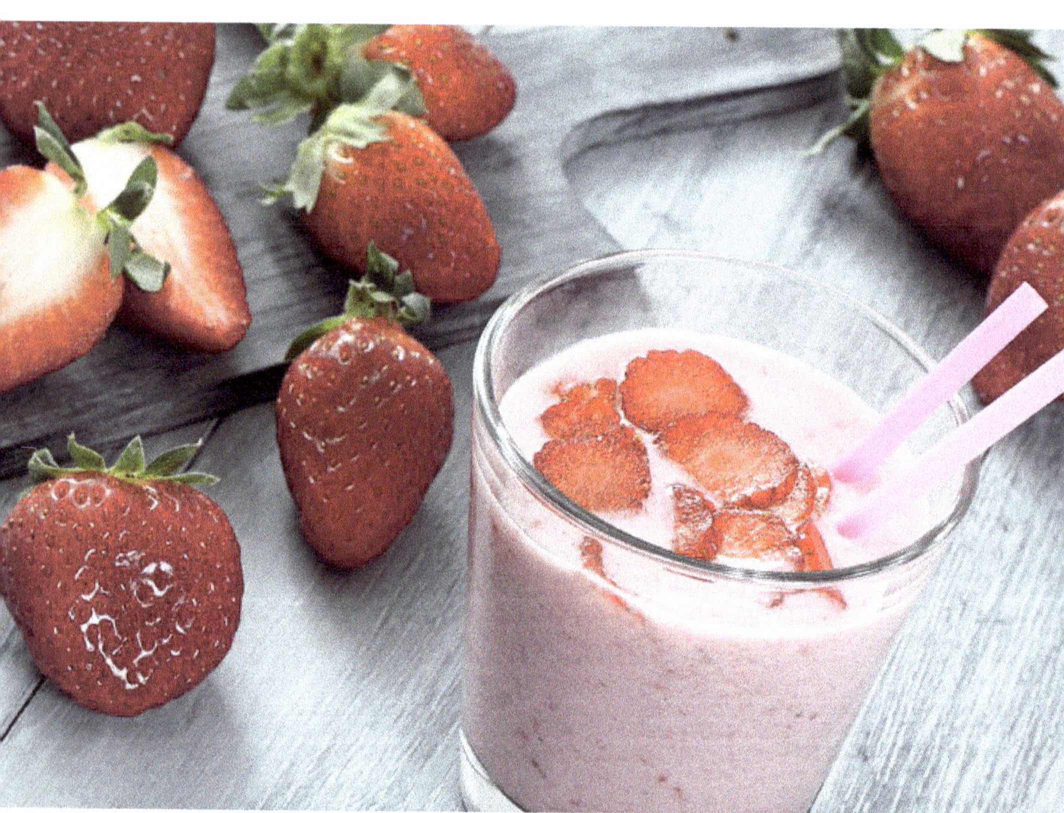

# Spiced Buttermilk

Preparation Time: 5 minutes | Cooking Time: 0 minute | Servings: 2

Ingredients:

- 3/4 teaspoon ground cumin
- 1/4 teaspoon sea salt
- 1/8 teaspoon ground black pepper
- 2 mint leaves
- 1/8 teaspoon lemon juice
- ¼ cup cilantro leaves
- 1 cup of chilled water
- 1 cup vegan yogurt, unsweetened
- Ice as needed

Directions:

- Place all the ingredients in the order in a food processor or blender, except for cilantro and ¼ teaspoon cumin, and then pulse for 2 to 3 minutes at high speed until smooth.

• Pour the milk into glasses, top with cilantro and cumin, and then serve.

Nutrition:

• Calories: 211 Total Carbohydrate: 7 g Cholesterol: 13 mg Total Fat: 18 g Fiber: 3 g Protein: 17 g Sodium: 289 mg

# Turmeric Lassi

Preparation Time: 5 minutes | Cooking Time: 0 minute | Servings: 2

Ingredients:

- 1 teaspoon grated ginger
- 1/8 teaspoon ground black pepper
- 1 teaspoon turmeric powder
- 1/8 teaspoon cayenne
- 1 tablespoon coconut sugar
- 1/8 teaspoon salt
- 1 cup vegan yogurt
- 1 cup almond milk

Directions:

- Place all the ingredients in the order in a food processor or blender and then pulse for 2 to 3 minutes at high speed until smooth.
- Pour the lassi into two glasses and then serve.

Nutrition:

- Calories: 392 Fat: 10g Protein: 18g Sugar: 8g

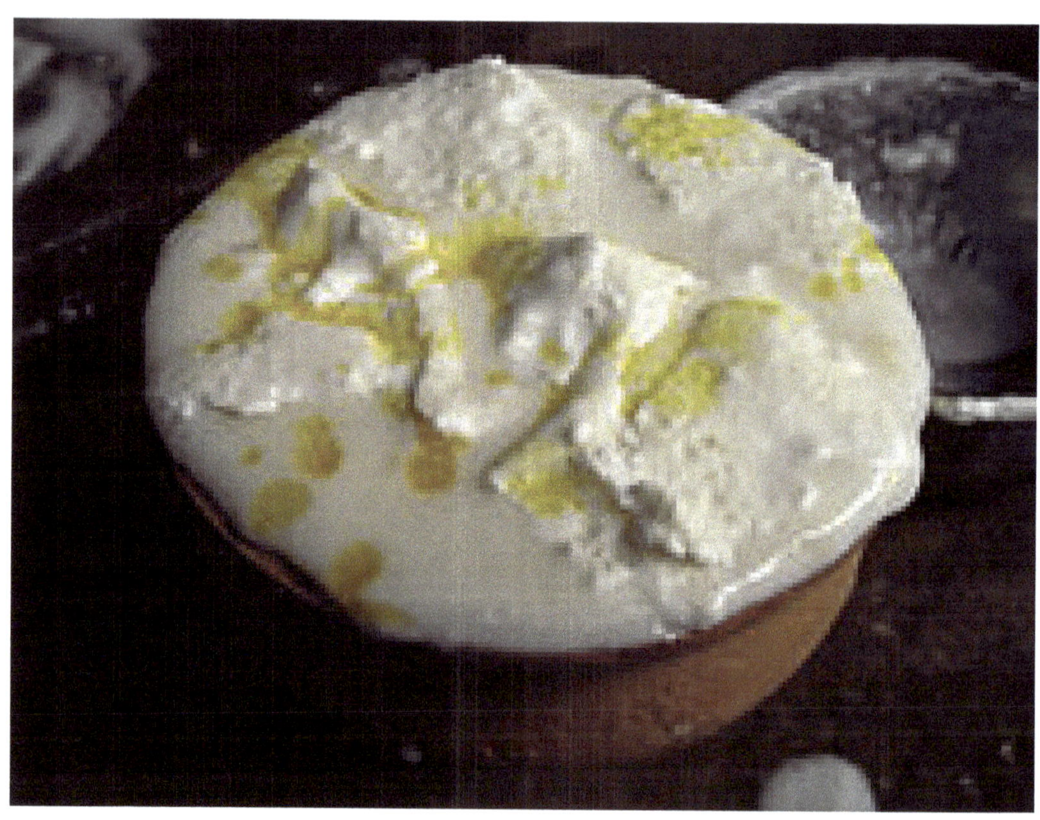

# Brownie Batter Orange Chia Shake

Preparation Time: 5 minutes | Cooking Time: 0 minute | Servings: 2

Ingredients:

- 2 tablespoons cocoa powder
- 3 tablespoons chia seeds
- ¼ teaspoon salt
- 4 tablespoons chocolate chips
- 4 teaspoons coconut sugar
- ½ teaspoon orange zest
- ½ teaspoon vanilla extract, unsweetened
- 2 cup almond milk

Directions:

- Place all the ingredients in the order in a food processor or blender and then pulse for 2 to 3 minutes at high speed until smooth.

• Pour the smoothie into two glasses and then serve.

Nutrition:

• Calories: 290 Fat: 11g Protein: 20g Sugar: 9g

# Saffron Pistachio Beverage

Preparation Time: 5 minutes | Cooking Time: 0 minute | Servings: 2

Ingredients:

- 8 strands of saffron

- 1 tablespoon cashews

- 1/4 teaspoon ground ginger

- 2 tablespoons pistachio

- 1/8 teaspoon cloves

- 1/4 teaspoon ground black pepper

- 1/4 teaspoon cardamom powder

- 3 tablespoons coconut sugar

- 1/4 teaspoon cinnamon

- 1/8 teaspoon fennel seeds

- 1/4 teaspoon poppy seeds

Directions:

- Place all the ingredients in the order in a food processor or blender and then pulse for 2 to 3 minutes at high speed until smooth.

• Pour the smoothie into two glasses and then serve.

Nutrition:

• Calories: 394 Fat: 5g Protein: 12g Sugar: 4g

# Mexican Hot Chocolate Mix

Preparation Time: 5 minutes | Cooking Time: 0 minute | Servings: 2

Ingredients:

- For the Hot Chocolate Mix:
- 1/3 cup chopped dark chocolate
- 1/8 teaspoon cayenne
- 1/8 teaspoon salt
- 1/2 teaspoon cinnamon
- 1/4 cup coconut sugar
- 1 teaspoon cornstarch
- 3 tablespoons cocoa powder
- 1/2 teaspoon vanilla extract, unsweetened
- For Servings:
- 2 cups milk, warmed

Directions:

- Place all the ingredients of the hot chocolate mix in the order in a food processor or blender and then pulse for 2 to 3 minutes at high speed until ground.

• Stir 2 tablespoons of the chocolate mix into a glass of milk until combined and then serve.

Nutrition:

• Calories: 160 Fat: 6g Protein: 26g Sugar: 7g

# Inspirational Orange Smoothie

Preparation Time: 5 minutes |

Cooking Time: 5 minutes |

Servings: 1

Ingredients:

- 4 mandarin oranges, peeled
- 1 banana, sliced and frozen
- ½ cup non-fat Greek yogurt
- ¼ cup of coconut water
- 1 tsp vanilla extract
- 5 ice cubes

Directions:

- Using a mixer, whisk all the ingredients.
- Enjoy your drink!

Nutrition:

- Calories 256 Fat 13.3 g Carbohydrates 0 g

Sugar 0 g Protein 34.5 g Cholesterol 78 mg

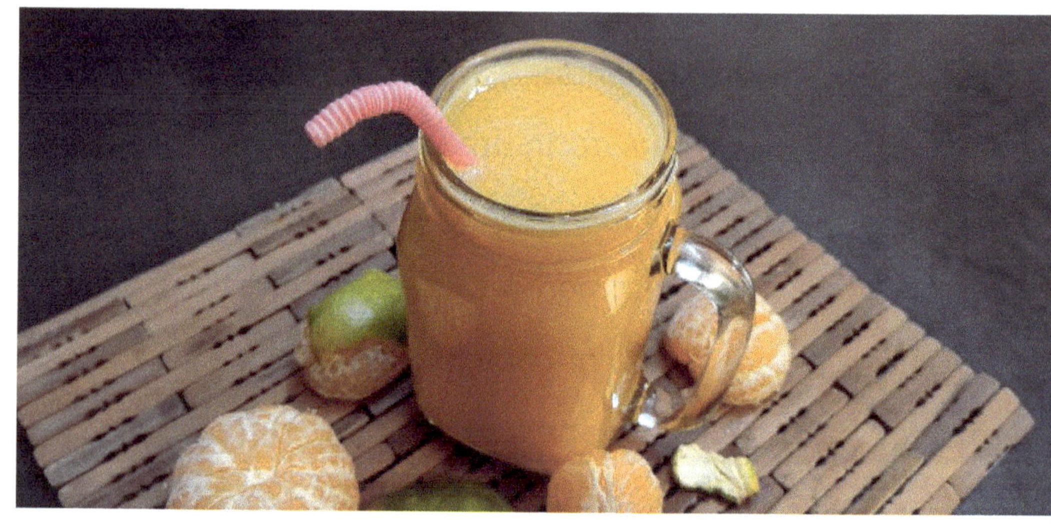

# High Protein Blueberry Banana Smoothie

Preparation Time: 5 minutes | Cooking Time: 5 minutes | Servings: 2

Ingredients:

- 1 cup blueberries, frozen
- 2 ripe bananas
- 1 cup of water
- 1 tsp vanilla extract
- 2 Tbsp chia seeds
- ½ cup cottage cheese
- 1 tsp lemon zest

Directions:

- Put all the smoothie ingredients into the blender and whisk until  smooth.
- Enjoy your wonderful smoothie!

Nutrition:

- Calories 358 Fat 19.8 g Carbohydrates 1.3 g Sugar 0.4 g Protein 41.9 g Cholesterol 131 mg

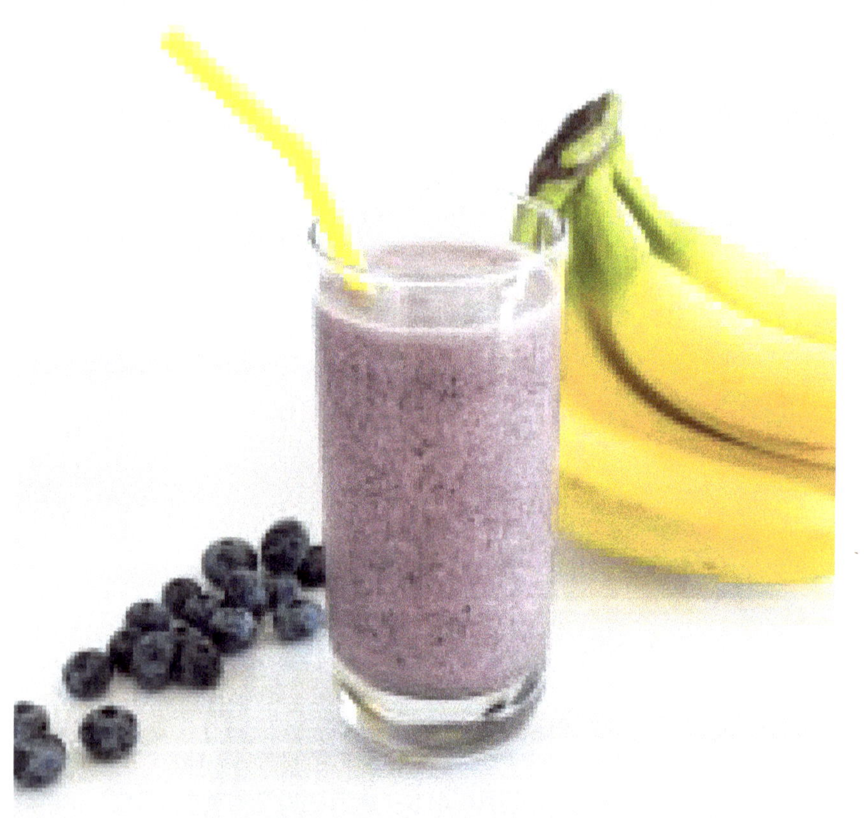

# Citrus Detox Juice

Preparation Time: 10 minutes | Cooking Time: 0 minutes | Servings: 4

Ingredients:

- Water (3 C.)

- Lemon (1, Sliced)

- Grapefruit (1, Sliced)

- Orange (1, Sliced)

Directions:

- Begin by peeling and slicing up your fruit. Once this is done, place it in a pitcher of water and infuse the water overnight.

Nutrition:

- Calories: 269 Total Carbohydrate: 2 g Cholesterol: 3 mg Total Fat: 14 g Fiber: 2 g Protein: 7 g Sodium: 183 mg

# Metabolism Water

Preparation Time: 10 minutes | Cooking Time: 0 minutes | Servings: 1

Ingredients:

* Water (3 C.)

* Cucumber (1, Sliced)

* Lemon (1, Sliced)

* Mint (2 Leaves)

* Ice

Directions:

* All you will have to do is get out a pitcher, place all of the ingredients in, and allow the ingredients to soak overnight for maximum benefits!

Nutrition:

* Calories: 301 Total Carbohydrate: 2 g Cholesterol: 13 mg Total Fat: 17 g Fiber: 4 g Protein: 8 g Sodium: 201 mg

# Stress Relief Detox Drink

Preparation Time: 5 minutes | Cooking Time: 0 minutes | Servings: 1

Ingredients:

- Water (1 Pitcher)

- Mint

- Lemon (1, Sliced)

- Basil

- Strawberries (1 C., Sliced)

- Ice

Directions:

- When you are ready, take all of the ingredients and place them into a pitcher of water overnight and enjoy the next day.

Nutrition:

- Calories: 189 Total Carbohydrate: 2 g Cholesterol: 73 mg Total Fat: 17 g Fiber: 0 g Protein: 7 g Sodium: 163 mg

# Strawberry Pink Drink

Preparation Time: 10 minutes | Cooking Time: 5 minutes | Servings: 4

Ingredients:

- Water (1 C., Boiling)
- Sugar (2 T.)
- Acai Tea Bag (1)
- Coconut Milk (1 C.)
- Frozen Strawberries (1/2 C.)

Directions:

- You will begin by boiling your cup of water and steep the teabag in for at least five minutes. • When the tea is set, add in the sugar and coconut milk. Be sure to stir well to spread the

sweetness throughout the tea.

- Finally, add in your strawberries, and you can

enjoy your freshly made pink drink! Nutrition:

- Calories: 321 Total Carbohydrate: 2 g

Cholesterol: 13 mg Total Fat: 17 g Fiber: 2 g

Protein: 9 g Sodium: 312 mg

# Lavender and Mint Iced Tea

• Preparation Time: 5 minutes | Cooking Time: 10 minutes | Servings: 8 servings

Ingredients:

- 8 cups of water

- 1/3 cup of dried lavender buds

- ¼ cup of mint

Directions:

- Add the mint and lavender to a pot and set this aside.

- Add eight cups of boiling water to the pot. Sweeten to taste, cover, and let steep for ten

minutes. Strain, chill and serve.

• Tips:

• Use a sweetener of your choice when making this iced tea.

- Add spirits to turn this iced tea into a summer cocktail.

Nutrition:

- Calories 266 Carbs: 9.3g Protein: 20.9g Fat: 16.1g

# Pear Lemonade

• Preparation Time: 5 minutes | Cooking Time: 30 minutes | Servings: 2 servings

Ingredients:

- ½ cup of pear, peeled and diced
- 1 cup of freshly squeezed lemon juice
- ½ cup of chilled water

Directions:

• Add all the ingredients into a blender and pulse until it has all been combined. The pear does make the lemonade frothy, but this will settle.

• Place in the refrigerator to cool and then serve.

• Tips:

• Keep stored in a sealed container in the refrigerator for up to four days.

• Pop the fresh lemon in the microwave for ten

minutes before juicing, you can extract more juice if you do this.

Nutrition:

- Calories: 160 Carbs: 6.3g Protein: 2.9g Fat: 13.6g

# Energizing Ginger Detox Tonic

Preparation Time: 15 minutes | Cooking Time: 10 minutes | Servings:

Ingredients:

- 1/2 teaspoon of grated ginger, fresh
- 1 small lemon slice
- 1/8 teaspoon of cayenne pepper
- 1/8 teaspoon of ground turmeric
- 1/8 teaspoon of ground cinnamon
- 1 teaspoon of maple syrup
- 1 teaspoon of apple cider vinegar
- 2 cups of boiling water

Directions:

• Pour the boiling water into a small saucepan, add and stir the ginger, then let it rest for 8 to

10 minutes, before covering the pan.

- Pass the mixture through a strainer and into the liquid, add the cayenne pepper, turmeric, cinnamon and stir properly.

- Add the maple syrup, vinegar, and lemon slice.

- Add and stir an infused lemon and serve immediately.

Nutrition:

- Calories 443 Carbs:9.7 g Protein: 62.8g Fat: 16.9g

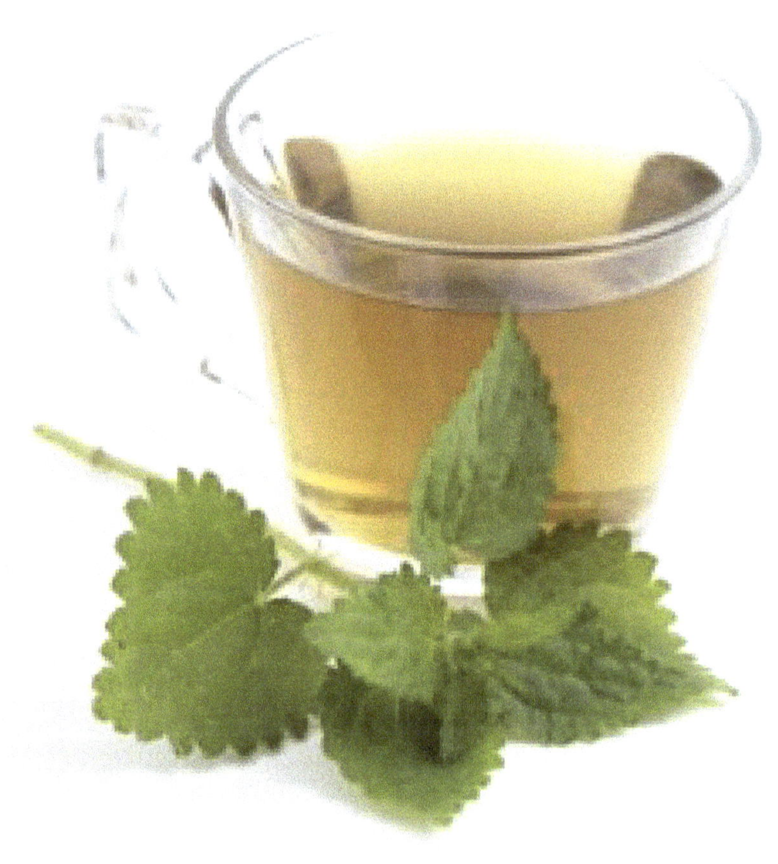

# Strawberry Shake

- Preparation Time: 10 minutes | Cooking Time: 10 minutes | Servings: 2

Ingredients:

- 1½ cups fresh strawberries, hulled
- 1 large frozen banana, peeled
- 2 scoops unsweetened vegan vanilla protein powder
- 2 tablespoons hemp seeds
- 2 cups unsweetened hemp milk

Directions:

- In a high-speed blender, place all the ingredients and pulse until creamy.
- Pour into two glasses and serve immediately.

Nutrition:

- Calories: 259 Fat: 3g Protein: 10g Sugar: 2g

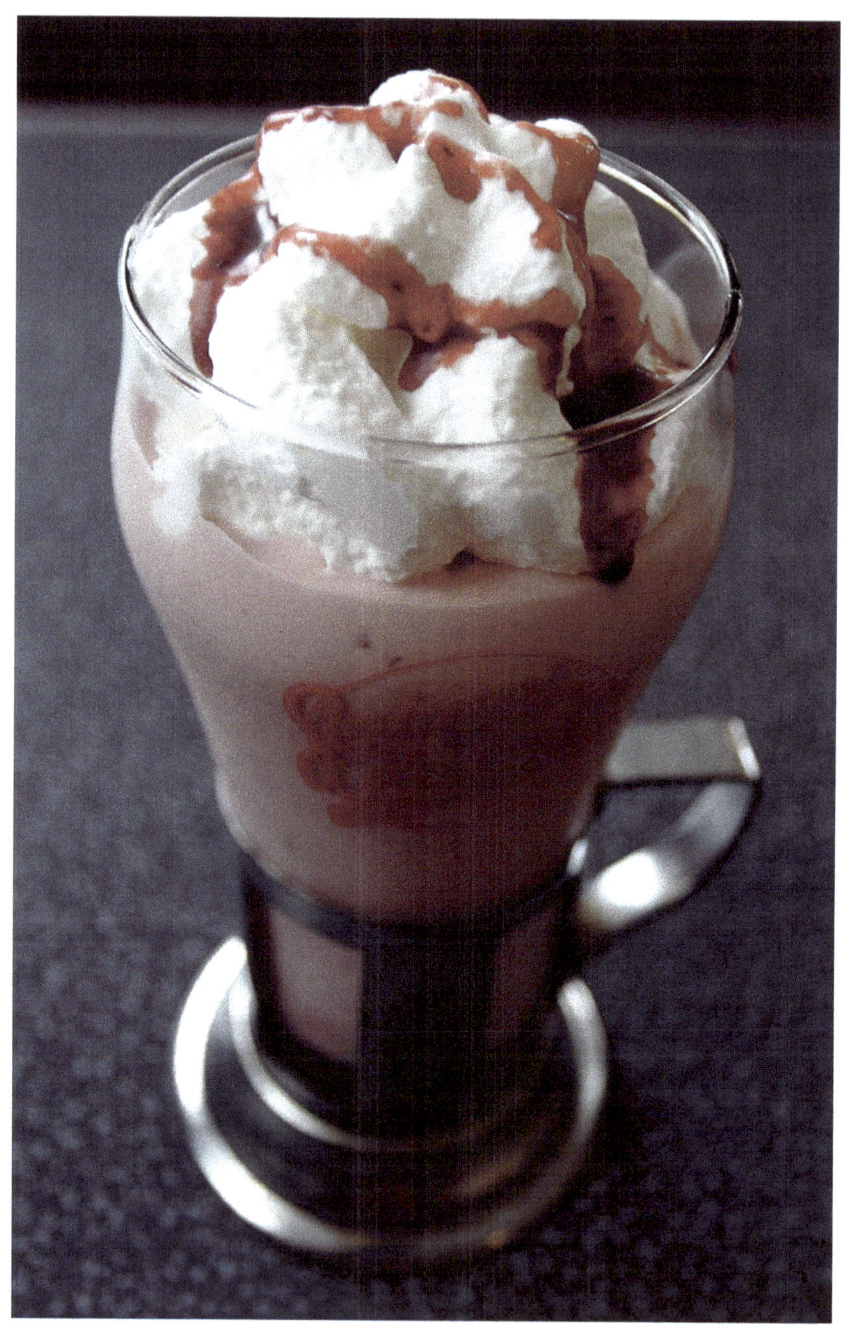

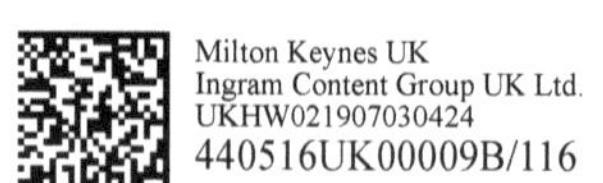
Milton Keynes UK
Ingram Content Group UK Ltd.
UKHW021907030424
440516UK00009B/116